# The Best Meat Recipes for Mum

*Easy and Tasty Recipes for Mediterranean Cookbook*

By Jasmine Mirrel

# Sommario

**We have actually gotten to completion of this wonderful yet tiny publication. I have actually presented you to my favorite dishes, however I'll maintain publishing even more publications with even more dishes. Make certain to exercise food preparation; attempt as well as attempt once again these scrumptious dishes that are healthy as well as healthy and balanced. Constantly speak to a medical professional prior to beginning any kind of dietary strategy and also take pleasure in life. I eagerly anticipate seeing you at the following one. Delight in.** ....................................................... 119

# Introduction

The Mediterranean Diet regimen comprises a collection of expertise as well as practices varying from landscape to table, consisting of plants, harvesting, angling, preservation, handling, prep work, and also intake of food.<br>

It is identified by a dietary version that has actually continued to be consistent in time as well as areas, being primarily comprised of: olive oil, grains, fresh as well as dried out fruits, veggies, a modest quantity of fish, milk items, meat, lots of flavorings, and also seasonings, completely accompanied by white wine. It is a design of a lasting diet plan, as it adds to maintain: top quality, food, and also dietary safety and security as well as at the same time advertises the administration of territorial as well as ecological sources.<br>

Mediterranean diet regimen is a particular diet regimen by getting rid of refined foods as well as high in saturated fats. It is regarding consuming typical active ingredients eaten by those that have actually lived in the Mediterranean container for a lengthy time. This is a diet regimen abundant in fruits, veggies, as well as fish.

# CHAPTER 1: MEAT RECIPES

## Lamb Vegetable Soup

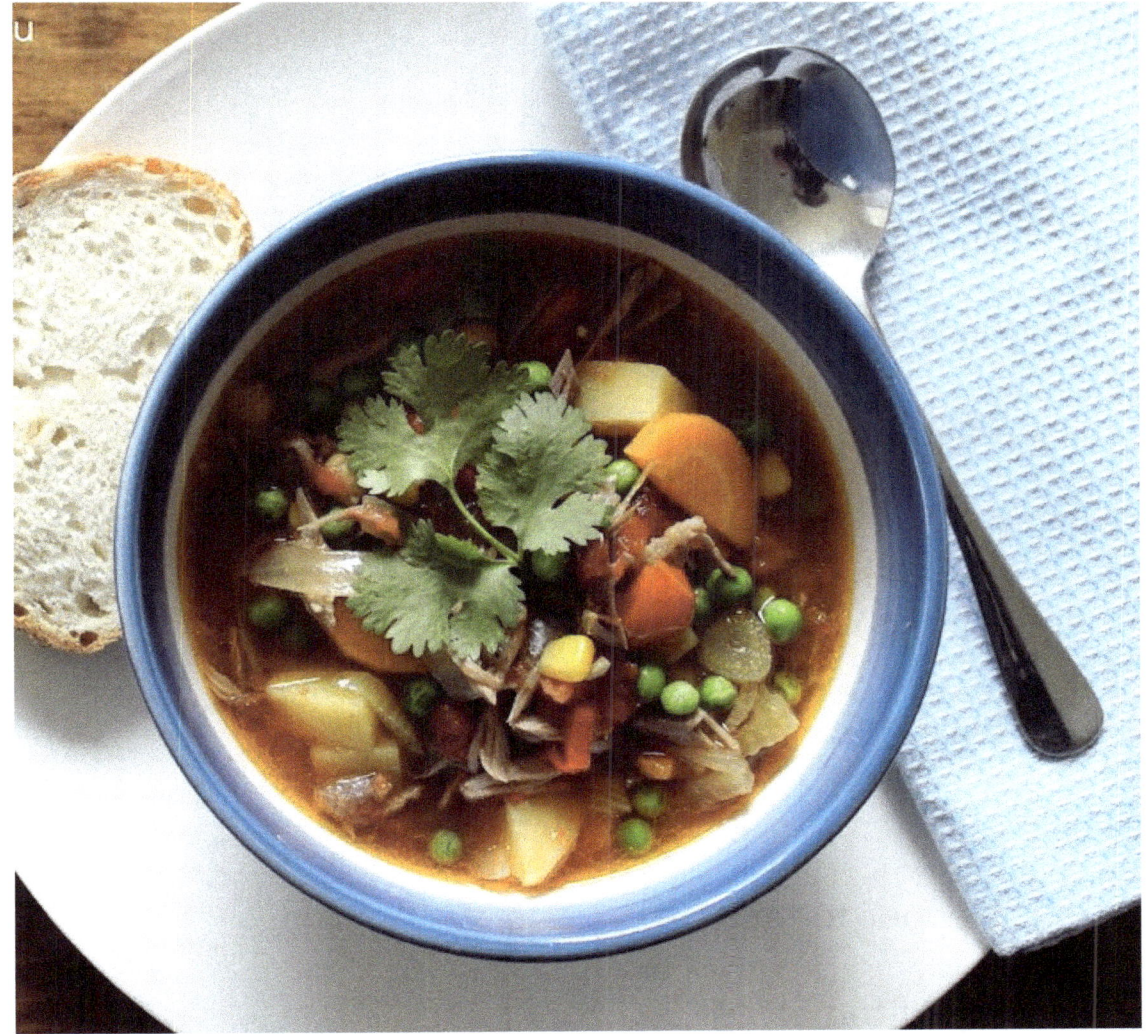

**Servings:** 8

**Preparation time:** 1 ½ Hour

### INGREDIENTS

- 1 ½ pound lamb shoulder, cubed

- 2 tablespoons olive oil

- 2 shallots, chopped

- 2 carrots. diced

- 2 celery stalks, diced

- ¼ teaspoon grated finger

- 2 cups cauliflower florets

- ½ cup green peas

- 4 cups vegetable stock

- 6 cups water

- 1 thyme spring

- 1 oregano spring

- 1 basil spring

- Salt and pepper to taste

- 1 can crushed tomatoes

- 2 tablespoons lemon juice

**DIRECTIONS**

1. Heat the oil in a soup pot and stir in the lamb shoulder.

2. Cook for some minutes on all sides, then add the water and stock.

3. Cook for 40 minutes, then add the rest of the ingredients and season with salt and pepper.

4. Continue cooking for another 20 minutes, then serve the soup fresh.

   **NUTRITION:** Calories 221, Fat 9,9g, Protein 25,7g, Carbs 6.5g

# Spanish Meatball Soup

**Servings:** 8

**Preparation time:** 1 Hour

## INGREDIENTS

- 2 tablespoons olive oil

- 1 onion, chopped

- 2 garlic cloves, chopped

- 2 red bell peppers, cored and diced

- 2 carrots. diced

- 1 celery stalk, diced

- 2 cups vegetable stock

- 6 cups enter

- 1 pound ground veal

- 1 egg

- 2 tablespoons chopped parsley

- 1 can crushed tomatoes

- Salt and pepper to taste

## DIRECTIONS

1. Heat the oil in a soup pot and stir in the onion, garlic, bell, peppers. carrots, celery stock, and water. Season with salt and pepper and bring to a boil.

2. In the meantime, mix the veal, egg, and parsley in a bowl. Form small meatballs and place them in the boiling liquid.

3. Add the tomatoes and adjust the taste with salt and pepper.

4. Cook on low heat for 20 minutes.

5. Serve the soup war and fresh.

   **NUTRITION:** Calories 166, Fat 8.5g, Protein: 15.6g, Carbs 6.5g

# Eggless Spinach & Bacon Quiche

**Servings:** 8

**Preparation time:** 20 minutes

## INGREDIENTS

1 cup fresh spinach, chopped

4 slices of bacon, cooked and chopped

½ cup mozzarella cheese. shredded

4 tablespoons milk

4 dashes Tabasco sauce

1 cup Parmesan cheese, shredded

Salt and freshly ground black pepper. to taste

## DIRECTIONS

1. Preheat the Airfryer to 325 degrees F and grease a baking dish.

2. Put all the ingredients in a bowl and mix well.

3. Transfer the mixture into a prepared baking dish and cook for about 8 minutes.

4. Dish out and serve.

**NUTRITION:** Calories 72, Carbs 0.9g, Fat 5,2g, Protein 5.5g, Sodium 271mg, Sugar: 0.4g

# Sausage & Bacon with Beans

**Servings:** 12

**Preparation time:** 30 Minutes

## INGREDIENTS

- 12 medium sausages

- 12 bacon slices

- 8 eggs

- 2 cans baked beans

- 12 bread slices, toasted

## DIRECTIONS

1. Preheat the Airfryer at 325 degrees F and place sausages and bacon in a fryer basket.

2. Cook for about 10 minutes and place the baked beans in a ramekin.

3. Place eggs in another ramekin and the Airfryer to 395 degrees F.

4. Cook for about 10 more minutes and divide the sausage mixture. beans and eggs in serving plates

5. Serve with bread slices.

**NUTRITION:** Calories 276, Carbs 14.1g, Fat 17g, Protein 16.3g, Sodium 817mg, Sugar: 0.6g

# Tomato-bacon Quiche

**Servings:** 6

**Preparation time:** 47 minutes

## INGREDIENTS

- 2 small medium-sized tomatoes, sliced

- ¼ tsp black pepper

- ¼ tsp salt

- ¼ tsp ground mustard

- ½ cup fresh spinach, chopped

- 2/4 cups cauliflower, ground into rice

- 5 slices nitrate-free bacon, cooked and chopped

- 3 tbsp unsweetened plain almond milk

- ½ cup organic white eggs

- 5 eggs, beaten

- 1/8 tsp sea salt

- 1 tbsp butter

- 1 tbsp flax meal

- 1 ½ tbsp coconut flour

- 1 egg, Beaten

- 2 small to medium-sized organic zucchini, grated

**DIRECTIONS**

1. Grease a pie dish and preheat the oven to 400 F.

2. Grate zucchini, drain, and squeeze dry.

3. In a bowl, add dry zucchini and remaining crust ingredients and mix well.

4. Place in the bottom of the pie plate and press down as if making a pie crust. Pop in the oven and bake for 9 minutes.

5. Meanwhile, in a large mixing bowl, whisk well black pepper, salt, mustard, almond milk, egg whites, and egg.

6. Add bacon, spinach, and cauliflower rice. Mix well. Pour into baked zucchini crust, top with tomato slices.

7. Pop back in the oven and bake for 28 minutes. If at 20 minutes baking time top is browning too much, cover with parchment paper for the remainder of cooking time.

8. Once done cooking, remove from oven, let it stand for at least ten minutes.

9. Slice into equal triangles, serve and enjoy.

**NUTRITION:** Calories 154, Protein 11.6g, Carbs 3.4g, Fat 10.3g

# Italian Meatball Soup

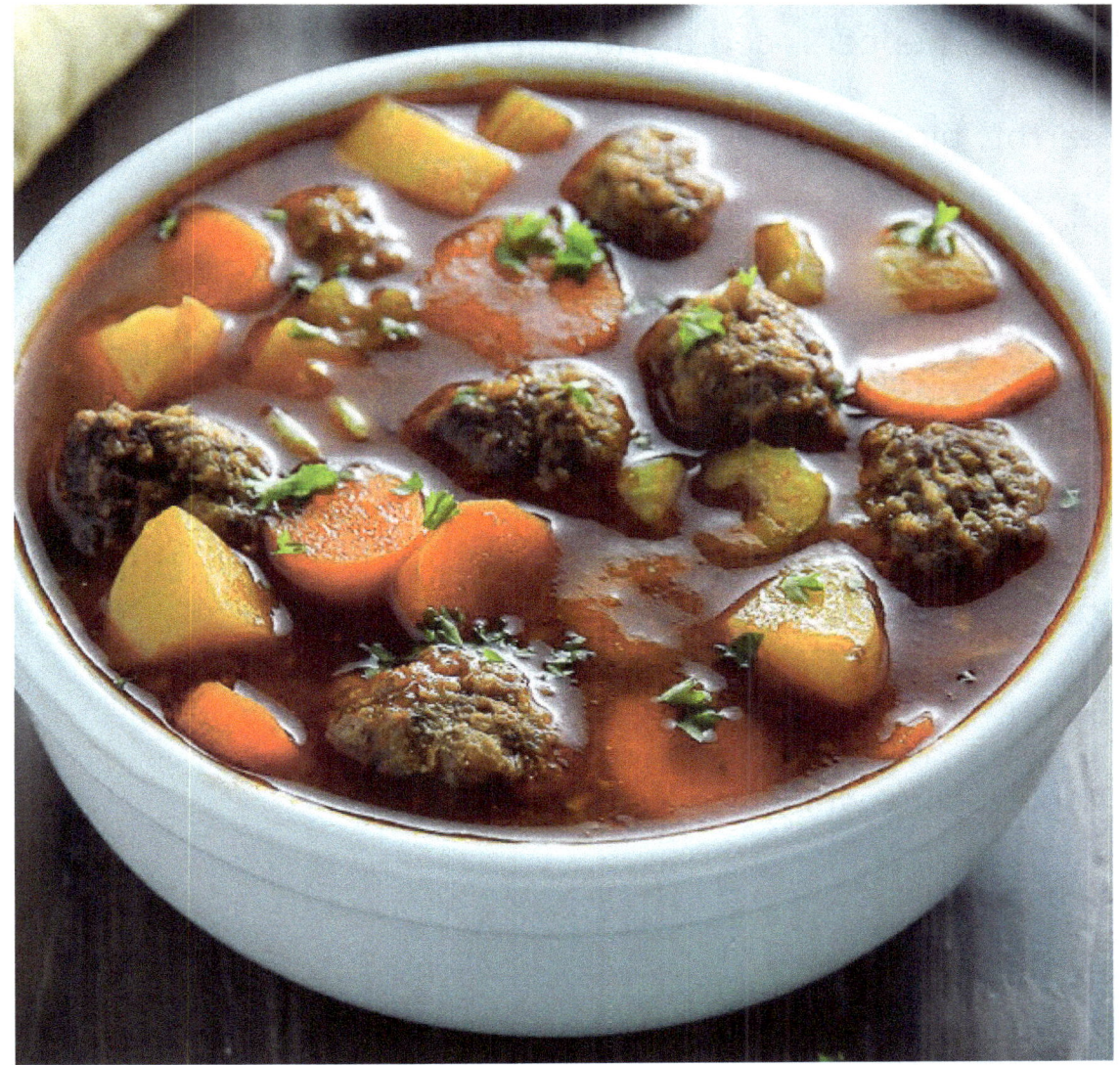

**Servings:** 8

**Preparation time:** 1 Hour

## INGREDIENTS

- 4 cups chicken stock

- 4 cups water

- 1 shallot, chopped

- 2 red bell peppers, cored and diced

- 1 carrot, diced

- 1 celery stalk, diced

- 2 tomatoes, diced

- 1 cup tomato juice

- ½ teaspoon dried oregano

- 1 teaspoon dried basil

- 1 pound ground chicken

- 2 tablespoons white rice

- 1 lemon, juiced

- Salt and pepper to taste

- 2 tablespoons chopped parsley

**DIRECTIONS**

Combine the stock, water, shallot, bell peppers, carrot, celery, tomatoes, tomato juice, oregano, and basil in a soup pot.

Add salt and pepper to taste and cook for 10 minutes.

Make the meatballs by mixing the chicken with rice and parsley.

Form small meatballs and drop them in the hot soup.

Continue cooking for another 15 minutes, then add the lemon

Serve the soup right away.

**NUTRITION:** Calories 150, Fat 4.7g, Protein 18g, Carbs 8.8g

# Meat Cakes

**Servings:** 4

**Preparation time:** 10 minutes

## INGREDIENTS

1 cup broccoli, shredded

½ cup ground pork

2 eggs, beaten

1 teaspoon salt

1 tablespoon Italian seasonings

1 teaspoon olive oil

3 tablespoons wheat flour, whole grain

1 tablespoon dried dill

## DIRECTIONS

In the mixing bowl, combine together shredded broccoli and ground pork.

Add salt, Italian seasoning, flour and dried dill.

Mix up the mixture until homogenous.

Then add eggs and stir until smooth.

Heat up olive oil in the skillet.

With the help of the spoon, make latkes and place them in the hot oil.

Roast the latkes for 4 minutes from each side over medium heat.

The cooked latkes should have a light brown crust.

Dry the latkes with paper towels if needed.

**NUTRITION:** Calories 143, Fat 6g, Fiber 0.9g, Carbs 7g, Protein 15.1g

# Moist Shredded Beef

**Servings:** 8

**Preparation time:** 30 minutes

## INGREDIENTS

- 2 lbs beef roast beef, cut into chunks

- ½ tbsp dried red pepper

- 1 tbsp Italian seasoning

- 1 tbsp garlic, minced

- 2 tbsp vinegar

- 14 oz can fire-roasted tomatoes

- ½ cup bell pepper, chopped

- ½ cup carrots, chopped

- 1 cup onion, chopped

- 1 tsp salt

## DIRECTIONS

Add all ingredients into the inner pot of the instant pot and set the pot on sauté mode.

Seal pot with lid and cook on high for 20 minutes.

Once done, release pressure using quick release.

Remove lid.

Shred the meat using a fork.

Stir well and serve.

**NUTRITION**: Calories 456, Fat 32.7g, Carbs 7.7g, Sugar 4.1g, Protein 31g, Cholesterol 118 mg

# Braised Beef In Oregano-Tomato Sauce

**Servings:** 12

**Preparation time:** 1 ½ Hour

## INGREDIENTS

- 2 onions, chopped

- 3 celery stalks, diced

- 4 cloves garlic, minced

- 2 (28-ounce) cans of Italian-style stewed tomatoes

- 1 cup dry red vine

- 1 teaspoon dried oregano

- 1 teaspoon salt

- 3 pounds boneless beef chuck roast, cut into 1-1/2 -inch cubes

- ½ cup chopped fresh parsley

- ¼ cup vegetable oil

- ¾ teaspoon black pepper

## DIRECTIONS

1. Place a pot on medium-high fire and heat for 2 minutes.

2. Add oil and heat for another 2 minutes.

3. Add beef and brown on all sides. Around 12 minutes.

4. Add onions, celery, and garlic, and sauté for 5 minutes or until vegetables are tender. Add remaining ingredients and bring to a boil.

5. Reduce heat to low, cover, and simmer for 60 minutes or until beef is fork-tender.

   **NUTRITION:** Calories 285, Carbs 7.4g, Protein 31.7g, Fat 14.6g

# Pork Chops And Herbed Tomato Sauce

**Servings:** 4

**Preparation time:** 10 minutes

## INGREDIENTS

4 pork loin chops, boneless

6 tomatoes, peeled and crushed

3 tablespoons parsley, chopped

2 tablespoons olive oil

¼ cup kalamata olives, pitted and halved

1 yellow onion, chopped

1 garlic clove, minced

## DIRECTIONS

1. Heat up a pan with the oil over medium heat, add the pork chops, cook them for 3 minutes on each side, and divide between plates.

2. Heat up the same pan again over medium heat, add the tomatoes, parsley, and the rest of the ingredients, whisk, simmer for 4 minutes, drizzle over the chops and serve.

**NUTRITION**: Calories 334, Fat 17g, Fiber 2g, Carbs 12g, Protein 34g

# Beef Shawarma

**Servings:** 2

**Preparation time:** 20 minutes

## INGREDIENTS

- ½ lb ground beef

- ¼ tsp cinnamon

- ½ tsp dried oregano

- 1 cup cabbage, cut into strips

- ½ cup bell pepper, sliced

- ¼ tsp ground coriander

- ½ tsp cumin

- ¼ tsp cayenne pepper

- ¼ tsp ground allspice

- ½ cup onion, chopped

- ½ tsp salt

## DIRECTIONS

1. Set instant pot on sauté mode.

2. Add meat to the pot and sauté until brown.

3. Add remaining ingredients and stir well.

4. Seal pot with lid and cook on high for 5 minutes.

5. Once done, release pressure using quick release. Remove lid.

6. Stir and serve.

**NUTRITION**: Calories 245, Fat 7.4g, Carbs 7.9g, Sugar 3.9g, Protein 35.6g, Cholesterol 101mg

# Beef Brisket And Veggies

**Servings:** 10

**Preparation time:** 4 Hours

## INGREDIENTS

- 3-pound beef brisket

- 1 carrot, peeled, chopped

- 1 onion, peeled

- 1 garlic clove, peeled

- 1 teaspoon peppercorns

- 1 teaspoon salt

- 1 teaspoon ground black pepper

- ½ bay leaf

- ½ cup crushed tomatoes

- 3 cups of water

- 1 celery stalk, chopped

## DIRECTIONS

1. Place the beef brisket in the saucepan.

2. Add carrot, onion, garlic clove, peppercorns, salt, ground black pepper, bay leaf, crushed tomatoes, celery stalk, and water.

3. Close the lid and bring the meat to a boil.

4. Simmer the meal for 4 hours over medium heat.

5. Serve the meat poached vegetables.

   **NUTRITION:** Calories 321, Fat 10.5g, Fiber 0.9g, Carbs 3g, Protein 50.4g

# Beef Curry

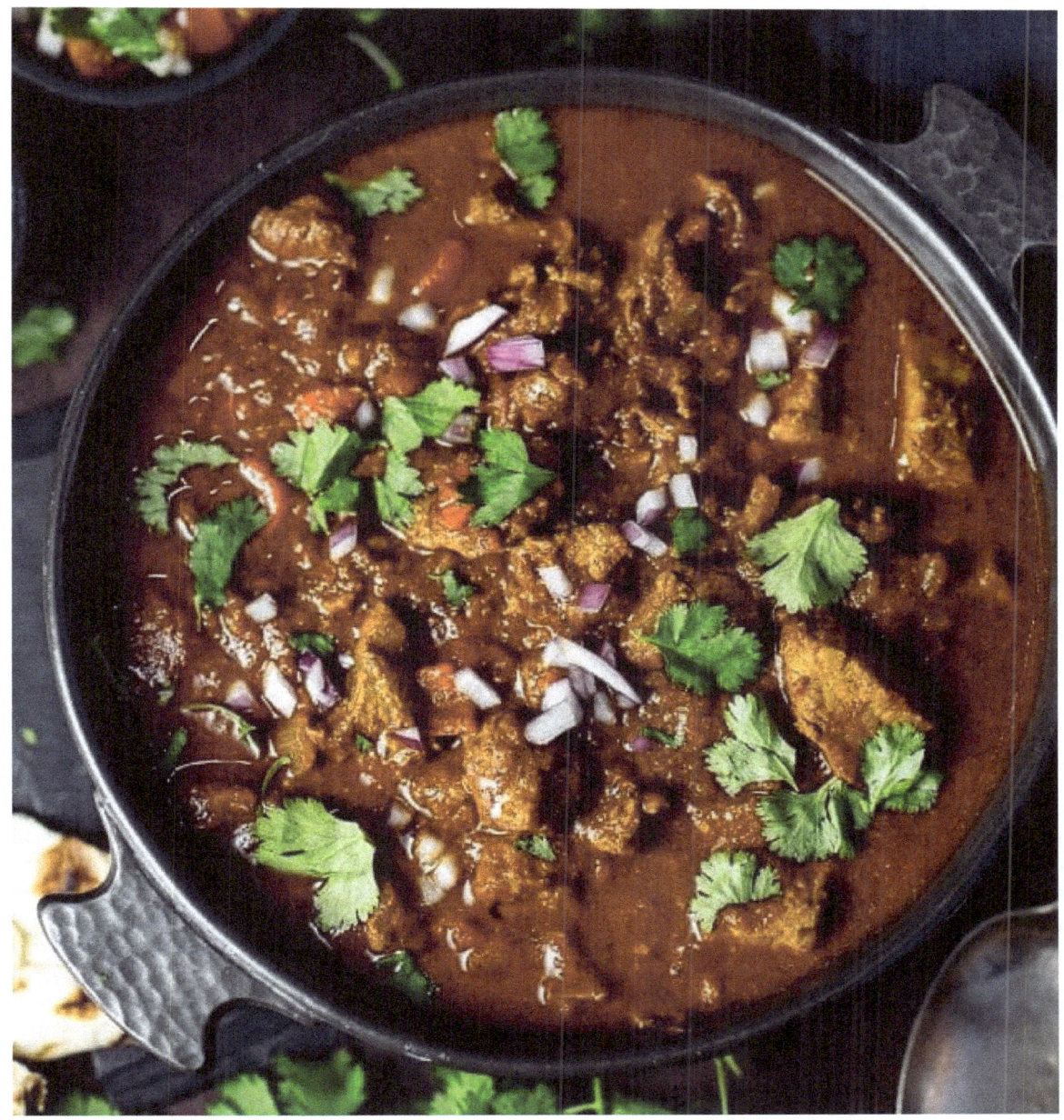

**Servings:** 2

**Preparation time:** 40 minutes

## INGREDIENTS

- ½ lb beef stew meat, cubed

- 1 bell peppers, sliced

- 1 cup beef stock

- 1 tbsp fresh ginger, grated

- ½ tsp ground cumin

- 1 tsp ground coriander

- ½ tsp cayenne pepper

- ½ cup sun-roasted tomatoes, diced

- 2 tbsp olive oil

- 1 tsp garlic, crushed

- 1 green chili peppers, chopped

## DIRECTIONS

1. Add all ingredients into the instant pot and stir well.

2. Seal pot with lid and cook on high for 30 minutes.

3. Once done, allow to release pressure naturally. Remove lid.

4. Serve and enjoy.

**NUTRITION**: Calories 391, Fat 21.9g, Carbs 11.6g, Sugar 5.8g, Protein 37.4g, Cholesterol 101mg

# Hearty Beef Ragu

**Servings:** 4

**Preparation time:** 1 hour

**INGREDIENTS**

- 1 ½ lbs beef steak. Diced

- 1 ½ cup beef stock

- 1 tbsp coconut amino

- 14 oz can tomatoes, chopped

- ½ tsp ground cinnamon

- 1 tsp dried oregano

- 1 tsp dried thyme

- 1 tsp dried basil

- 1 tsp paprika

- 1 bay leaf

- 1 tbsp garlic, chopped

- ½ tsp cayenne pepper

- 1 celery stick, diced

- 1 carrot, diced

- 1 onion, diced

- 2 tbsp olive oil

- ¼ tsp pepper

- 1 ½ tsp sea salt

**DIRECTIONS**

1. Add oil into the instant pot and set the pot on sauté mode.

2. Add celery, carrots, onion, and salt and sauté for 5 minutes.

3. Add meat and remaining ingredients and stir everything well.

4. Seal pot with lid and cook on high for 30 minutes.

5. Once done, allow to release pressure naturally for 10 minutes, then release remaining using quick release. Remove lid.

6. Shred meat using a fork. Set pot on sauté mode and cook for 10 minutes. Stir every 2-3 minutes.

7. Serve and enjoy.

**NUTRITION**: Calories 435, Fat 18.1g, Carbs 12.3g, Sugar 5.5g, Protein 54.4g, Cholesterol 152mg

# Hot Pork Meatballs

**Servings:** 2

**Preparation Time:** 10 minutes

## INGREDIENTS

- 4 oz pork loin, grinded

- ½ teaspoon garlic powder

- ¼ teaspoon chili powder

- ¼ teaspoon cayenne pepper

- ¼ teaspoon ground black pepper

- ¼ teaspoon white pepper

- 1 tablespoon water

- 1 teaspoon olive oil

## DIRECTIONS

1. Mix up together garlic powder, cayenne pepper, ground black pepper, white pepper, and water.

2. With the help of the fingertips, make the small meatballs.

3. Heat up olive oil in the skillet.

4. Range in the oil and cook for 10 minutes totally. Flip on another side from time to time.

   **NUTRITION**: Calories 162, Fat 10.3g, Fiber 0.3g, Carbs 1g, Protein 15.7g

# Beef And Zucchini Skillet

**Servings:** 2

**Preparation time:** 20 minutes

## INGREDIENTS

- 2 oz ground beef

- ½ onion, sliced

- ½ bell pepper, sliced

- 1 tablespoon butter

- ½ teaspoon salt

- 1 tablespoon tomato sauce

- 1 small zucchini, chopped

- ½ teaspoon dried oregano

## DIRECTIONS

1. Place the ground beef in the skillet.

2. Add salt, butter, and dried oregano.

3. Mix up the meat mixture and cook it for 10 minutes.

4. After this, transfer the cooked ground beef to the bowl.

5. Place zucchini, bell pepper, and onion in the skillet (where the ground meat was cooking) and roast the vegetables for 7 minutes over medium heat or until they are tender.

6. Then add cooked ground beef and tomato sauce. Mix up well.

7. Cook the beef toss for 2-3 minutes over medium heat.

**NUTRITION:** Calories 182, Fat 8.7g, Fiber 0.1g, Carbs 0.3g, Protein 24.1g

# Meatloaf

**Servings:** 6

**Preparation time:** 35 minutes

## INGREDIENTS

2 lbs ground beef

2 eggs, lightly beaten

¼ tsp dried basil

3 tbsp olive oil

½ tsp dried sage

1 ½ tsp dried parsley

1 tsp oregano

1 tsp thyme

1 tsp rosemary

Pepper

Salt

## DIRECTIONS

Pour 1 ½ cups of water into the instant pot, then place the trivet in the pot.

Spray loaf pan with cooking spray.

Add all ingredients into the mixing bowl and mix until well combined.

Transfer meat mixture into the prepared loaf pan and place loaf pan on top of the trivet in the pot.

Seal pot with lid and cook on high for 35 minutes.

Once done, allow to release pressure naturally for 10 minutes, then release remaining using quick release. Remove lid.

Serve and enjoy.

**NUTRITION:** Calories 365, Fat 18g, Carbs 0.7g, Sugar 0.1g, Protein 47.8g, Cholesterol 190mg

# Tasty Lamb Ribs

**Servings:** 4

**Preparation time:** 2 Hours

## INGREDIENTS

- 2 garlic cloves, minced

- ¼ cup shallot, chopped

- 2 tablespoons fish sauce

- ½ cup veggie stock

- 2 tablespoons olive oil

- 1 and ½ tablespoons lemon juice

- 1 tablespoon coriander seeds, ground

- 1 tablespoon ginger, grated

- Salt and black pepper to the taste

- 2 pounds lamb ribs

## DIRECTIONS

1. In a roasting pan, combine the lamb with the garlic, shallots, and the rest of the ingredients, toss, introduce in the oven at 300 degrees F and cook for 2 hours.

2. Divide the lamb between plates and serve with a side salad.

**NUTRITION:** Calories 293, Fat 9.1g, Fiber 9.6g, Carbs 16.7g, Protein 2402g

# Peas And Han Thick Soup

**Servings:** 4

**Preparation time:** 30 minutes

## INGREDIENTS

- Pepper and salt to taste

- 1 lb. Ham, coarsely chopped

- 24 oz frozen sweet peas

- 4 cup ham stock

- ¼ cup white wine

- 1 carrot, chopped coarsely

- 1 onion, chopped coarsely

- 2 tbsp butter, divided

## DIRECTIONS

1. On a medium pot, heat oil. Sauté for 6 minutes the onion or until soft and translucent.

2. Add wine and cook for 4 minutes or until nearly evaporated.

3. Add ham stock and bring to a simmer and simmer continuously while covered for 4 minutes.

4. Add peas and cook for 7 minutes or until tender.

5. Meanwhile, in a nonstick fry pan, cook to a bronzed crisp the ham in 1 tbsp butter, around 6 minutes. Remove from fire and set aside.

6. When peas are soft, transfer to a blender and puree. Return to pot, continue cooking while seasoning with pepper, salt, and ½ of crisped ham. Once the soup is to your desired taste, turn off the fire.

7. Transfer to 4 serving bowls and garnish evenly with crisped ham.

   **NUTRITION:** Calories 403, Carbs: 32.5g, Protein 32.5g, Fat 12.5g

# Garlic Caper Beef Roast

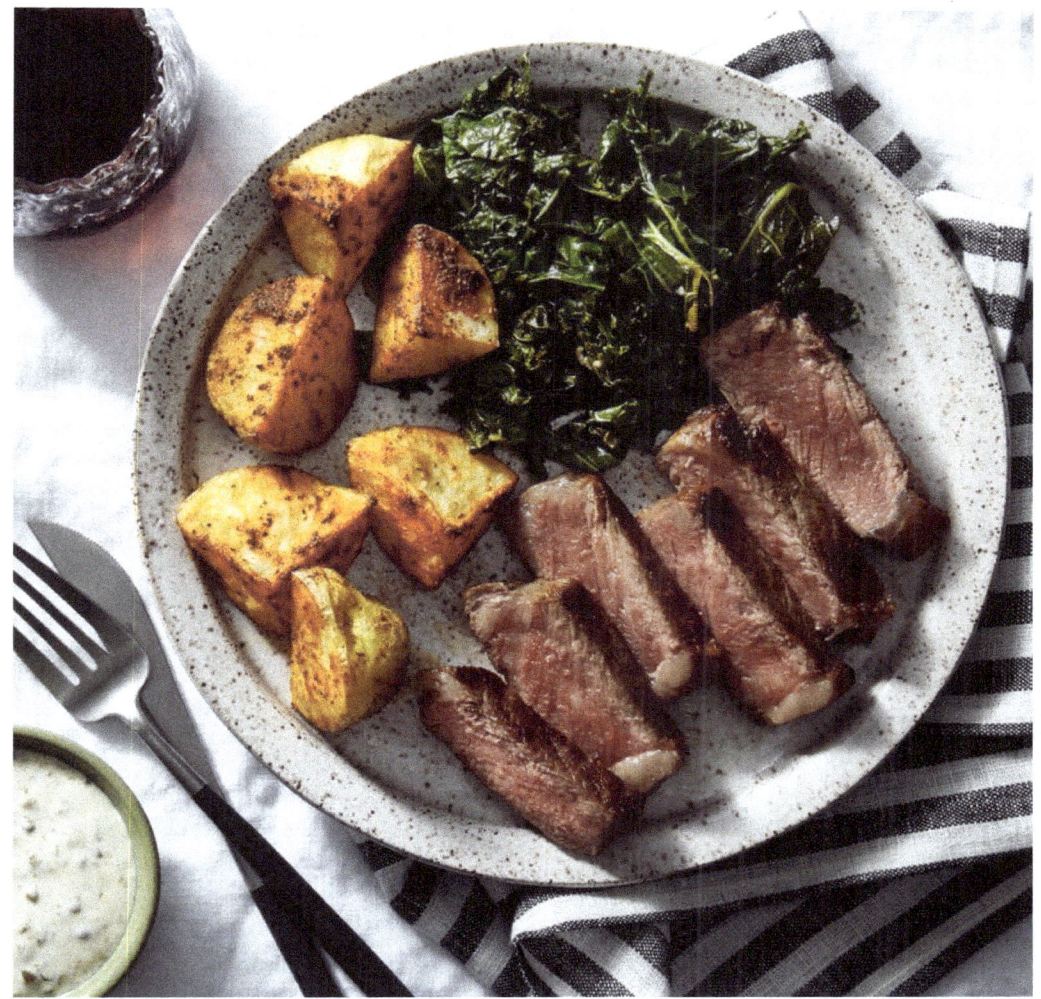

**Servings:** 4

**Preparation time:** 40 minutes

## INGREDIENTS

- 2 lbs beef roast, cubed

- 1 tbsp fresh parsley, chopped

- 1 tbsp capers, chopped

- 1 tbsp garlic, minced

- 1 cup chicken stock

- ½ tsp dried rosemary

- ½ tsp ground cumin

- 1 onion, chopped

- 1 tbsp olive oil

- Pepper

- Salt

## DIRECTIONS

1. Add oil into the instant pot and set the pot on sauté mode.

2. Add garlic and onion and sauté for 5 minutes.

3. Add meat and cook until brown.

4. Add remaining ingredients and stir well.

5. Seal pot with lid and cook on high for 30 minutes.

6. Once done, allow to release pressure naturally. Remove lid. Stir well and serve.

**NUTRITION:** Calories 470, Carbs 3.9g, Sugar 1.4g, Protein 69.5g, Cholesterol 203mg

# Beef Spread

**Servings:** 4

**Preparation time:** 25 minutes

**INGREDIENTS**

- 8 oz beef liver

- ½ onion, peeled

- ½ carrot, peeled

- ½ teaspoon peppercorns

- 1 bay leaf

- ½ teaspoon salt

- 1/3 cup water

- 1 teaspoon ground black pepper

**DIRECTIONS**

1. Chop the beef liver and put it in the saucepan.

2. Add onion, carrot, peppercorns, bay leaf, salt, and ground black pepper.

3. Add water and close the lid.

4. Boil the beef liver for 25 minutes or until all ingredients are tender.

5. Transfer the cooked mixture to the blender and blend it until smooth.

6. Then place the cooked pate in the serving bowl and flatten the surface of it.

7. Refrigerate the pate for 20-30 minutes before serving.

**NUTRITION:** Calories 109, Fat 2.7g, fiber 0.6g, Carbs 5.3g, Protein 15.3g

# Pork Chops And Relish

**Servings:** 6

**Preparation time:** 14 minutes

## INGREDIENTS

- 6 pork chops, boneless

- 7 ounces marinated artichoke hearts, chopped and their liquid reserved

- A pinch of salt and black pepper

- 1 teaspoon hot pepper sauce

- 1 and ½ cups tomatoes, cubed

- 1 jalapeno pepper, chopped

- ½ cup roasted bell peppers, chopped

- ½ cup black olives, pitted and sliced

## DIRECTIONS

1. In a bowl, mix the chops with the pepper sauce, reserved liquid from the artichokes, cover, and keep in the fridge for 15 minutes.

2. Heat up a grill over medium-high heat, add the pork chops and cook for 7 minutes on each side.

3. In a bowl, combine the artichokes with the peppers and the remaining ingredients, toss, divide on top of the chops and serve.

**NUTRITION:** Calories 215, Fat 6g, Fiber 1g, Carbs 6g, Protein 35g

# Tasty Beef Goulash

**Servings:** 2

**Preparation time:** 30 minutes

## INGREDIENTS

½ lb beef stew meat, cubed

1 tbsp olive oil

½ onion, chopped

½ cup sun-dried tomatoes, chopped

¼ zucchini, chopped

½ cabbage, sliced

1 ½ tbsp olive oil

2 cups chicken broth

Pepper

Salt

## DIRECTIONS

1. Add oil into the instant pot and set the pot on sauté mode.

2. Add onion and sauté for 3-5 minutes.

3. Add tomatoes and cook for 5 minutes.

4. Add remaining ingredients and stir well.

5. Seal pot with lid and cook on high for 20 minutes.

6. Once done, allow to release pressure naturally for 10 minutes, then release remaining using quick release. Remove lid.

7. Stir well and serve.

**NUTRITION:** Calories 389, Fat 15.8g, Carbs 19.3g, Sugar 10.7g, Protein 43.2g, Cholesterol 101mg

# Pork and Prunes Stew

**Servings:** 8

**Preparation time:** 1 ¼ Hours

**INGREDIENTS**

2 pounds pork tenderloin, cubed

2 tablespoons olive oil

1 Sweet onion, chopped

4 garlic cloves, chopped

2 carrots, diced

2 celery stalks, chopped

2 tomatoes, peeled and diced

1 cup vegetable stock

½ cup white wine

1 pound prunes, pitted

1 bay leaf

1 thyme spring

1 teaspoon mustard seeds

1 teaspoon coriander seeds

Salt and pepper to taste

## DIRECTIONS

1. Combine all the ingredients in a deep dish baking pan.

2. Add salt and pepper to taste and cook in the preheated oven at 350F for 1 hour, adding more liquid as it cooks if needed.

3. Serve and stew warm and fresh.

   **NUTRITION:** Calories 363, Fat 7.9g, Protein 31.7g, Carbs 41.4g

# Pork And Rice Soup

**Servings:** 4

**Preparation time:** 7 Hours

## INGREDIENTS

- 2 pounds pork stew meat, cubed

- A pinch of salt and black pepper

- 6 cups water

- 1 leek, sliced

- 1 bay leaves

- 1 carrot, sliced

- 3 tablespoons olive oil

- 1 cup white rice

- 2 cups yellow onion, chopped

- ½ cup lemon juice

- 1 tablespoon cilantro, chopped

## DIRECTIONS

In your slow cooker, combine the pork with the water and the rest of the ingredients except the cilantro, put the lid on, and cook on Low for 7 hours.

Stir the soup, ladle into bowls, sprinkle the cilantro on top, and serve.

**NUTRITION:** Calories 300, Fat 15g, Fiber 7.6g, Carbs 17.4g, Protein 22.4g

# Sage Pork And Beans Stew

**Servings:** 4

**Preparation time:** 4 Hours and 10 minutes

## INGREDIENTS

- 2 pounds pork stew meat, cubed

- 2 tablespoons olive oil

- 1 Sweet onion, chopped

- 1 red bell pepper, chopped

- 3 Garlic cloves, minced

- 2 teaspoons sage, dried

- 4 ounces canned white beans, drained

- 1 cup beef stock

- 2 zucchinis, chopped

- 2 tablespoons tomato paste

- 1 tablespoon cilantro, chopped

## DIRECTIONS

1. Heat up a pan with the oil over medium-high heat, add the meat, brown for 10 minutes, and transfer to your slow cooker.

2. Add the rest of the ingredients except the cilantro, put the lid on, and cook on High for 4 hours.

3. Divide the stew into bowls, sprinkle the cilantro on top, and serve

   **NUTRITION:** Calories 423, Fat 15.4g, Fiber 9.6g, Carbs 2704g, Protein 43g

# Pear Braised Pork

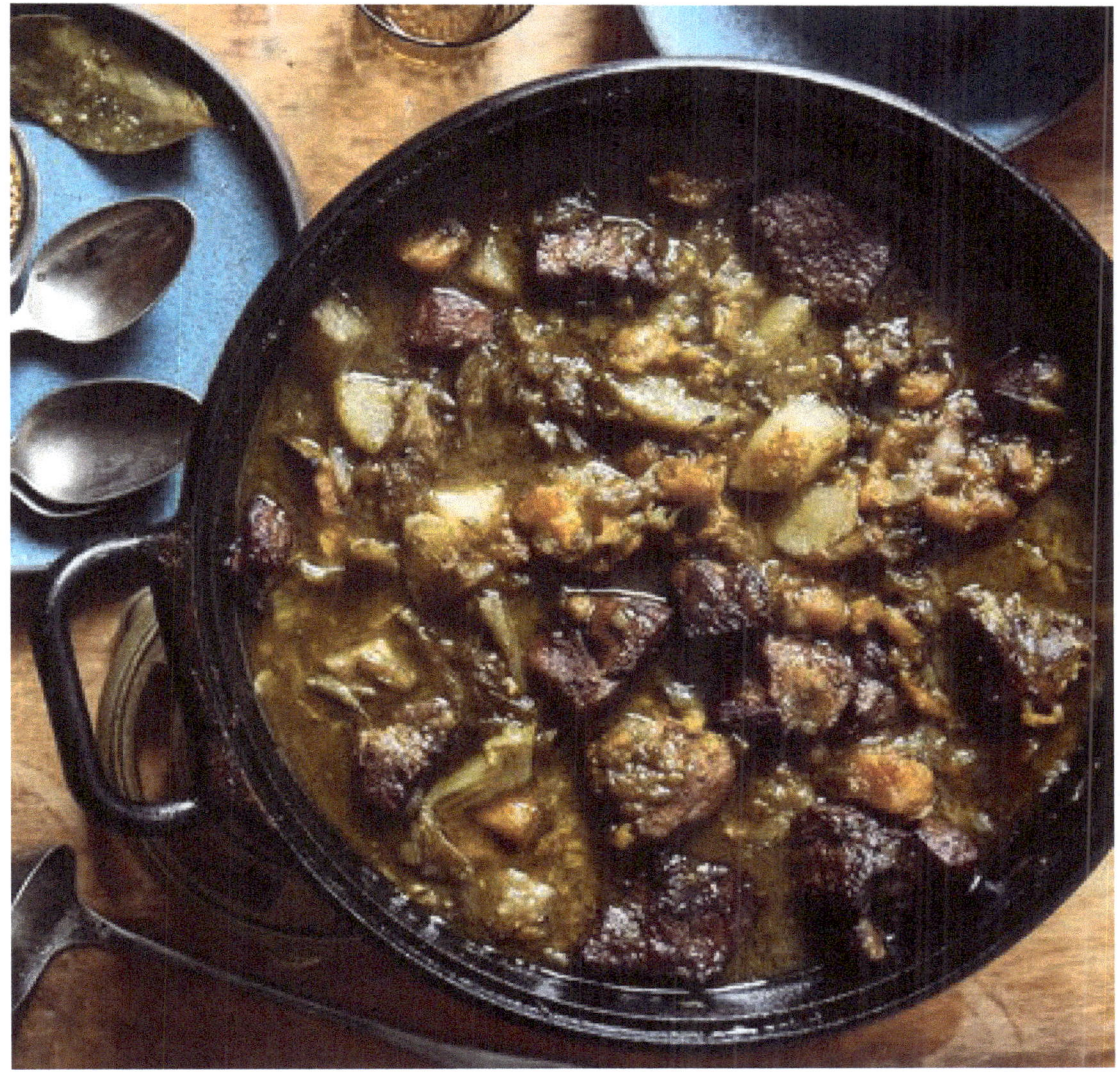

**Servings**: 10

**Preparation time:** 2 ¼ hours

## INGREDIENTS

- 3 pounds pork shoulder

- 4 Pears, peeled and sliced

- 2 shallots, sliced

- 4 garlic cloves, minced

- 1 bay leaf

- 1 thyme spring

- ½ cup apple cider

- Salt and pepper to taste

## DIRECTIONS

1. Season the pork with salt and pepper.

2. Combine the pears, shallots, garlic, bay leaf, thyme, and apple cider in a deep dish baking pan.

3. Place the pork over the pears, then cover the pan with aluminum foil.

4. Cook in the preheated oven at 330F for 2 hours. Serve the pork and the sauce fresh.

   **NUTRITION:** Calories 455, Fat 29.3g, Protein 32.1g, Carbs 14.9g

# Tasty Beef Stew

**Servings:** 4

**Preparation time:** 30 minutes

## INGREDIENTS

2 ½ lbs beef roast, cut into chunks

1 cup beef broth

½ cup balsamic vinegar

1 tbsp honey

½ tsp red pepper flakes

1 tbsp garlic, minced

Pepper

Salt

## DIRECTIONS

1. Add all ingredients into the inner pot of the instant pot and stir well.

2. Seal pot with lid and cook on high for 30 minutes.

3. Once done, allow to release pressure naturally. Remove lid.

4. Stir well and serve.

**NUTRITION:** Calories 562, Fat 18g, Carbs 5.7g, Sugar 4.6g, Protein 87.5g, Cholesterol 253mg

# Pork And Sage Couscous

**Servings:** 4

**Preparation time:** 7 Hours

## INGREDIENTS

- 2 pounds pork loin boneless and sliced

- ¾ cup veggie stock

- 2 tablespoons olive oil

- ½ tablespoon chili powder

- 2 teaspoon sage, dried

- ½ tablespoon garlic powder

- Salt and black pepper to the taste

- 2 cups couscous, cooked

## DIRECTIONS

In a slow cooker, combine the pork with the stock and the other ingredients except for the couscous, put the lid on, and cook on low for 7 hours.

Divide the mix between plates, add the couscous on the side, sprinkle the sage on top, and serve.

**NUTRITION:** Calories 270, Fat 14.5g, Fiber 9g, Carbs 16.3g, Protein 14.3g

# Beef And Potatoes With Tahini Sauce

**Servings:** 1/6 Casserole

**Preparation time:** 35 minutes

## INGREDIENTS

½ large yellow onion

1 lb. ground beef

½ tsp. salt

½ tsp. ground black pepper

6 small red potatoes, washed

3 TB. extra-virgin olive oil

2 cups plain Greek yogurt

¾ cup tahini paste

1½ cups water

¼ cup fresh lemon juice

1 TB. minced garlic

½ cup pine nuts

## DIRECTIONS

Preheat the oven to 425°F.

In a food processor fitted with a chopping blade, blend yellow onion for 30 seconds.

Transfer onion to a large bowl. Add beef, 1 teaspoon salt, black pepper, and mix well.

Spread beef mixture evenly in the bottom of a 9-inch casserole dish, and bake for 20 minutes.

Cut red potatoes into 1/4-inch-thick pieces, place in a bowl, and toss with 2 tablespoons extra-virgin olive oil and ½ teaspoon salt.

Spread potatoes on a baking sheet and bake for 20 minutes.

In a large bowl, combine Greek yogurt, tahini paste, water, lemon juice, garlic, and the remaining 1 teaspoon salt.

Remove beef mixture and potatoes from the oven. Using a spatula, transfer potatoes to the casserole dish. Pour yogurt sauce over the top and bake for 15 more minutes.

In a small pan over low heat, heat the remaining 1 tablespoon extra- virgin olive oil. Add pine nuts and toast for 1 or 2 minutes.

Remove casserole dish from the oven, spoon pine nuts over the top and serve warm with brown rice.

**NUTRITION** Calories 342, Fat 11g, Protein 31g, Carbs 30g, Fiber 6g

# Spicy Beef Chili Verde

**Servings:** 2

**Preparation time:** 23 minutes

## INGREDIENTS

- ½ lb beef stew meat, cut into cubes

- ¼ tsp chili powder

- 1 tbsp olive oil

- 1 cup chicken broth

- 1 Serrano pepper. chopped

- 1 tsp garlic, minced

- 1 small onion, chopped

- ½ cup grape tomatoes, chopped

- ½ cup tomatillos, chopped

- Pepper

- Salt

## DIRECTIONS

Add oil into the instant pot and set the pot on sauté mode.

Add garlic and onion and sauté for 3 minutes. Add remaining ingredients and stir well.

Seal pot with lid and cook on high for 20 minutes. Once done, allow to release pressure naturally. Remove lid.

Stir well and serve.

**NUTRITION:** Calories 317, Fat 15g, Carbs 6.4g, Sugar 2.6g, Protein 37g, Cholesterol 100mg

# Coriander Pork And Chickpeas Stew

**Servings:** 4

**Preparation Time:** 8 Hours

## INGREDIENTS

- ½ cup beef stock

- 1 tablespoon ginger, grated

- 1 teaspoon coriander. ground

- z teaspoons cumin, ground

- Salt and black pepper to the taste

- 2 and ½ pounds pork stew meat, cubed

- 28 ounces canned tomatoes, drained and chopped

- 1 red onion, chopped

- 4 garlic cloves, minced

- ½ cup apricots, cut into quarters

- 15 ounces canned chickpeas, drained

- 1 tablespoon cilantro, chopped

## DIRECTIONS

In your slow cooker, combine the meat with the stock, ginger, and the rest of the ingredients except the cilantro and the chickpeas, put the lid on, and cook on Low for 7 hours and 40 minutes.

Add the cilantro and the chickpeas, cook the stew on low for 20 minutes more, divide into bowls and serve.

**NUTRITION**: Calories 283, Fat 11.9g, Fiber 4.5g, Carbs 28.8g, Protein 25.4g

# Yogurt Marinated Pork Chops

**Servings:** 6

**Preparation time:** 2 Hours

## INGREDIENTS

6 pork chops

1 cup plain yogurt

1 mandarin, sliced

2 garlic cloves, chopped

1 red pepper, chopped

Salt and pepper to taste

## DIRECTIONS

1. Season the pork with salt and pepper and mix it with the remaining ingredients in a zip lock bag.

2. Marinate for 1 ½ hours in the fridge.

3. Heat a grill pan over medium flame and cook the pork chops on each side until browned.

4. Serve the pork chops fresh and warm.

**NUTRITION**: Calories 293, Fat 20.4g, Protein 20.6g, Carbs 4.4g

# Beef And Grape Sauce

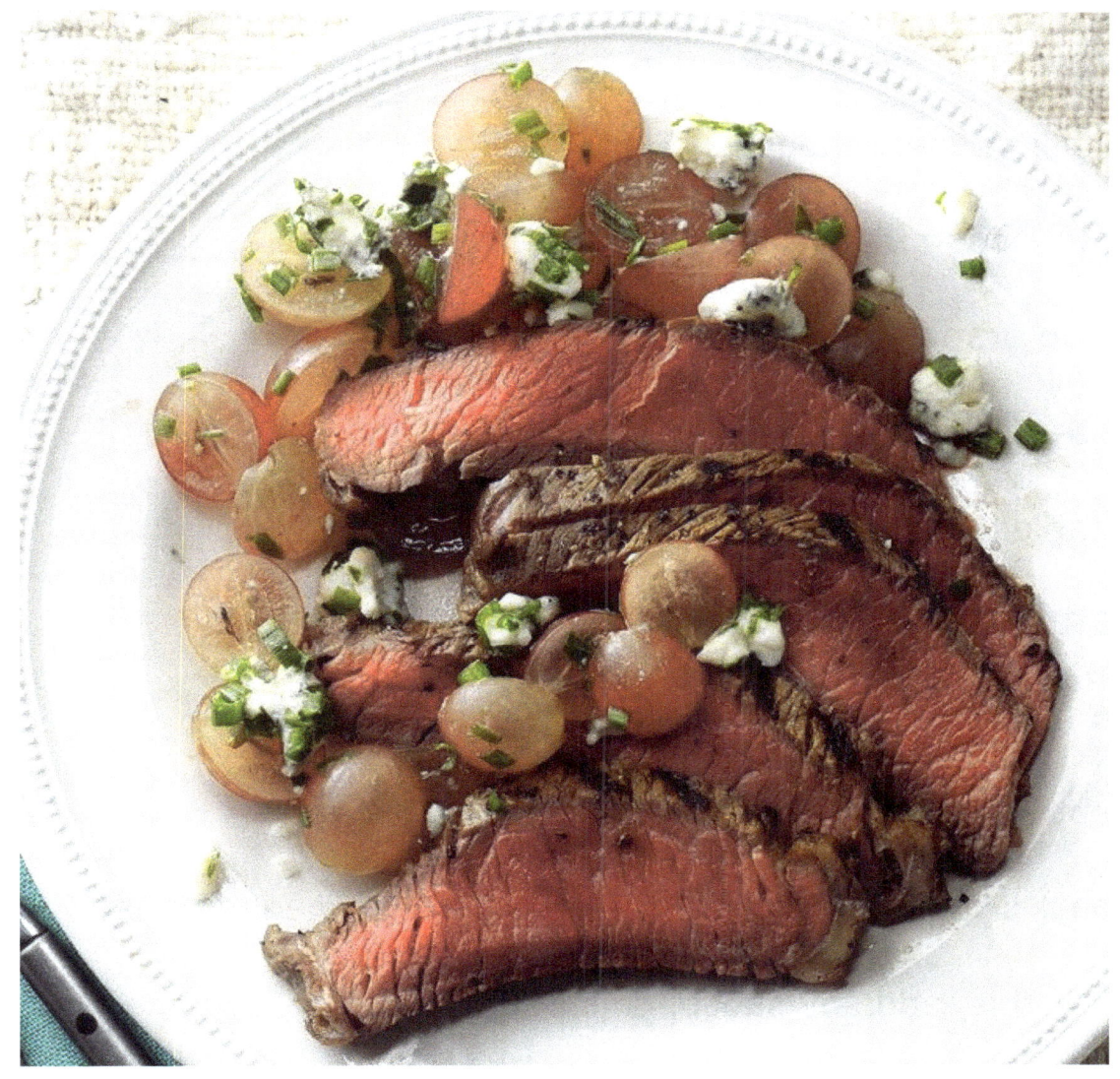

**Servings:** 4

**Preparation time:** 25 minutes

**INGREDIENTS**

- 1-pound beef sirloin

- 1 teaspoon molasses

- 1 tablespoon lemon zest, grated

- 1 teaspoon soy sauce

- 1 chili pepper, chopped

- ¼ teaspoon fresh ginger, minced

- 1 cup grape juice

- ½ teaspoon salt

- 1 tablespoon butter

## DIRECTIONS

1. Sprinkle the beef sirloin with salt and minced ginger.

2. Heat up butter in the saucepan and add meat.

3. Roast it for 5 minutes from each side over medium heat.

4. After this, add soy sauce, chili pepper, and grape juice.

5. Then add lemon zest and simmer the meat for 10 minutes.

6. Add molasses and mix up meat well.

7. Close the lid and cook meat for 5 minutes.

8. Serve the cooked beef with grape juice sauce.

**NUTRITION:** Calories 267, Fat 10g, Fiber 0.2g, Carbs 7.4g, Protein 34.9g

# Lamb And Tomato Sauce

**Servings:** 3

**Preparation time:** 55 minutes

## INGREDIENTS

- 9 oz lamb shanks

- 1 onion, diced

- 1 carrot, diced

- 1 tablespoon olive oil

- 1 teaspoon salt

- 1 teaspoon ground black pepper

- 1 ½ cup chicken stock

- 1 tablespoon tomato paste

## DIRECTIONS

Sprinkle the lamb shanks with salt and ground black pepper.

Heat up olive oil in the saucepan.

Add lamb shanks and roast them for 5 minutes from each side.

Transfer meat to the plate.

After this, add onion and carrot to the saucepan.

Roast the vegetables for 3 minutes.

Add tomato paste and mix up well.

Then add chicken stock and bring the liquid to a boil.

Add lamb shanks, stir well and close the lid.

Cook the meat for 40 minutes over medium-low heat.

**NUTRITION:** Calories 232, Fat 11.3g, Fiber 1.7g, Carbs 7g, Protein 25g

# Lamb And Sweet Onion Sauce

**Servings:** 4

**Preparation time:** 40 minutes

## INGREDIENTS

- 2 pounds lamb meat, cubed

- 1 tablespoon sweet paprika

- Salt and black pepper to the taste

- 1 and ½ cups veggie stock

- 4 garlic cloves, minced

- 2 tablespoons olive oil

- 1 pound sweet onion, chopped

- 1 cup balsamic vinegar

## DIRECTIONS

1. Heat up a pot with the oil over medium heat, add the onion, vinegar. salt and pepper, stir, and cook for 10 minutes.

2. Add the meat and the rest of the ingredients. Toss, bring to a simmer, and cook over medium heat for 30 minutes.

3. Divide the mix between plates and serve.

**NUTRITION:** Calories 303, Fat 12.3g, Fiber 7g, Carbs 15g, Protein 17g

# Pork And Mustard Shallots Mix

**Servings:** 4

**Preparation time:** 25 minutes

## INGREDIENTS

3 shallots, chopped

1 pound pork loin, cut into strips

½ cup veggie stock

2 tablespoons olive oil

A pinch of salt and black pepper

2 teaspoons mustard

1 tablespoon parsley, chopped

## DIRECTIONS

Heat up a pan with the oil over medium-high heat, add the shallots and sauté for 5 minutes.

Add the meat and cook for 10 minutes tossing it often.

Add the rest of the ingredients, toss, cook for 10 minutes more, divide between plates and serve right away.

**NUTRITION:** Calories 296, Fat 12.5g, Fiber 9.3g, Carbs 13.3g, Protein 22.5g

# Basil And Shrimp Quinoa

**Servings:** 1 Cup

**Preparation time:** 20 minutes

**INGREDIENTS**

3 TB. extra-virgin olive oil

2 TB. minced garlic

1 cup fresh broccoli florets

3 stalk asparagus, chopped

4 cups chicken or vegetable broth

½ tsp. salt

1 tsp. ground black pepper

1 TB. lemon zest

2 cups red quinoa

½ cup fresh basil, chopped

**DIRECTIONS**:

1. ½ lb. medium raw shrimp (18 to 20), shells and veins removed

2. In a 2-quart pot over low heat, heat extra-virgin olive oil. Add garlic and cook for 3 minutes.

3. Increase heat to medium, add broccoli and asparagus, and cook for 2 minutes.

4. Add chicken broth, salt, black pepper, lemon zest, and bring to a boil. Stir in red quinoa, cover, and cook for 15 minutes.

5. Fold in basil and shrimp, cover, and cook for 10 minutes.

6. Remove from heat, fluff with a fork, cover, and set aside for 10 minutes. Serve warm.

   **NUTRITION** Calories 128, Fat 12g, Fiber 6g, Protein 29g, Carbs 18g

# Ground Pork Salad

**Servings:** 8

**Preparation time:** 15 minutes

## INGREDIENTS

- 1 cup ground pork

- ½ onion, diced

- 4 bacon slices

- 1 teaspoon sesame oil

- 1 teaspoon butter

- 1 cup lettuce, chopped

- 1 tablespoon lemon juice

- 4 eggs, boiled

- ½ teaspoon salt

- 1 teaspoon chili pepper

- ¼ teaspoon liquid honey

## DIRECTIONS

1. Make burgers: in the mixing bowl, combine together ground pork, diced onion, salt, and chili pepper.

2. Blake the medium size burgers.

3. Melt butter in the skillet and add prepared burgers.

4. Roast them for 5 minutes from each side over medium heat.

5. When the burgers are cooked, chill them a little.

6. Place the bacon in the skillet and roast it until golden brown. Then chill the bacon and chop it roughly.

7. In the salad bowl, combine together chopped bacon, sesame oil, lettuce, lemon juice, and honey. Mix up salad well.

8. Peel the eggs and cut them on the halves.

9. Arrange the eggs and burgers over the salad. Don't mix salad anymore.

   **NUTRITION:** Calories 213, Fat 15.5g, Fiber 0.1g, Carbs 1.5g, Protein 16.5g

# Beef And Dill Mushrooms

**Servings:** 3

**Preparation time:** 35 minutes

## INGREDIENTS

1 cup cremini mushrooms, sliced

4 oz beef loin, sliced onto the wedges

1 tablespoon olive oil

1 teaspoon dried oregano

½ cup of water

¼ cup cream

1 teaspoon tomato paste

1 teaspoon ground black pepper

1 teaspoon salt

1 tablespoon fresh dill, chopped

## DIRECTIONS

In the saucepan, combine together olive oil and cremini mushrooms.

Add dried oregano, ground black pepper, salt and dill. Mix up.

Cook the mushrooms for 2-3 minutes and add sliced beef loin.

Cook the ingredients for 5 minutes over medium heat.

After this, add cream, water, tomato paste, and mix up the meal

Simmer the beef stroganoff for 25 minutes over the medium heat

**NUTRITION:** Calories 196, Fat 11.8g, Fiber 0.8g, Carbs 3.5g, Protein 20g

# Beef Pitas

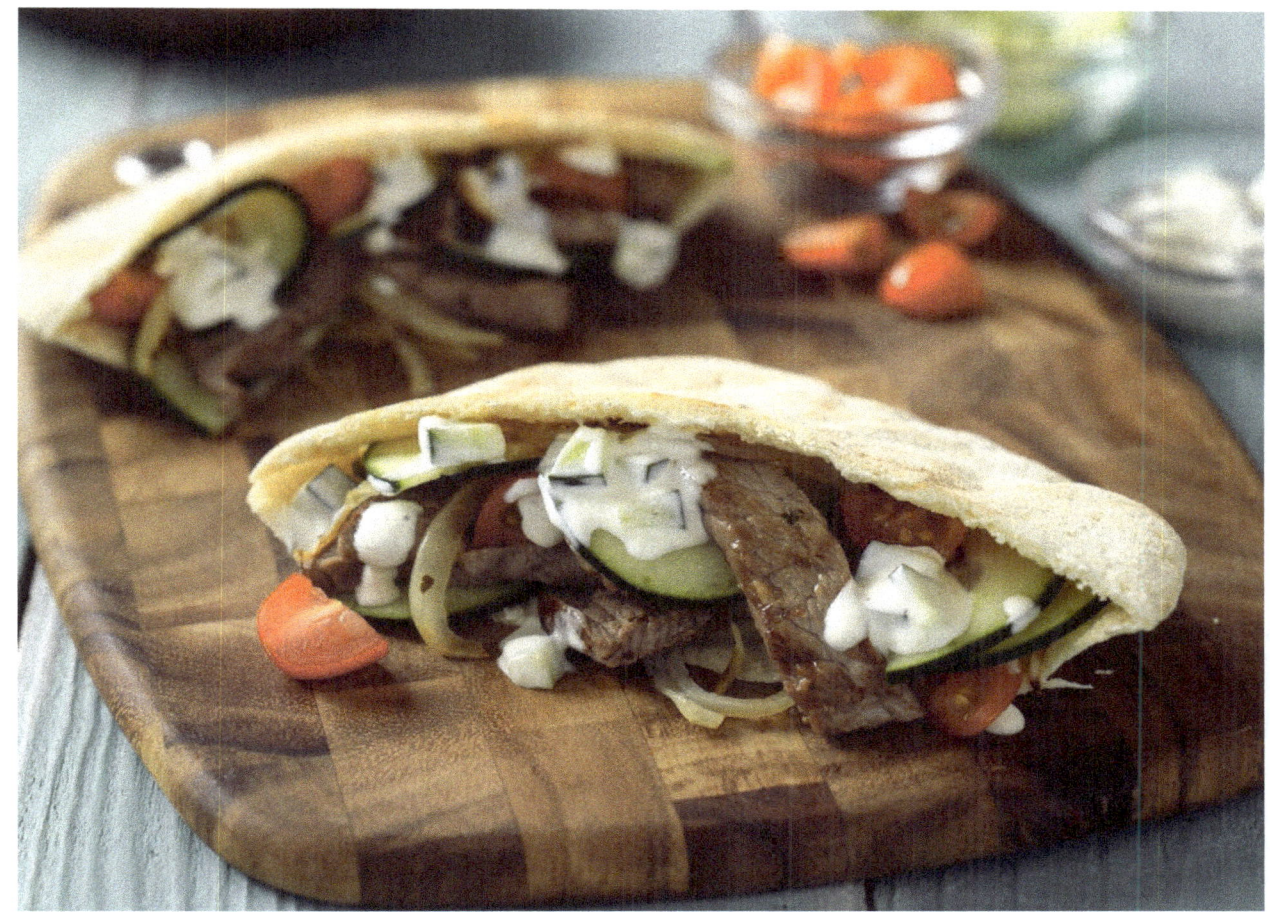

**Servings:** 4

**Preparation time:** 15 minutes

## INGREDIENTS

- 1 ½ cup ground beef

- ½ red onion, diced

- 1 teaspoon minced garlic

- ¼ cup fresh spinach, chopped

- 1 teaspoon salt

- ½ teaspoon chili pepper

- 1 teaspoon dried oregano

- 1 teaspoon fresh mint, chopped

- 4 tablespoons Plain yogurt

- 1 cucumber, grated

- ½ teaspoon dill

- ½ teaspoon garlic powder

- 4 pitta bread

## DIRECTIONS

1. In the mixing bowl, combine together ground beef, onion, minced garlic, spinach, salt, chili pepper, and dried oregano.

2. Blake the medium size balls from the meat mixture.

3. Line the baking tray with baking paper and arrange the meatballs inside.

4. Bake the meatballs for 15 minutes at 375F. Flip them on another side after 10 minutes of cooking.

5. Meanwhile, make tzatziki: combine together fresh mint, yogurt, grated cucumber, dill, and garlic powder. Whisk the mixture for 1 minute.

6. When the meatballs are cooked, place the over pitta bread and top with tzatziki.

   **NUTRITION:** Calorie 253, Fat 7g, Fiber 4g, Carbs 30g, Protein 16.3g

# Rosemary Lamb

**Servings:** 4

**Preparation time:** 6 Hours

## INGREDIENTS

- 2 pounds lamb shoulder, cubed

- 1 tablespoon rosemary, chopped

- 3 garlic cloves, minced

- ½ cup lamb stock

- 4 bay leaves

- Salt and black pepper to the taste

## DIRECTIONS

1. In your slow cooker. combine the lamb with the rosemary and the rest of the ingredients. put the lid on and cook on High for 6 hours.

2. Divide the mix between palates and serve.

**NUTRITION:** Info: Calories 290, Fat 13g, Fiber 11.6g, Carbs 18.3g, Protein 14g

# Rosemary Creamy Beef

**Servings:** 4

**Preparation time:** 50 minutes

## INGREDIENTS

2 lbs beef stem meat. cubed

2 tbsp fresh parsley, chopped

1 tsp garlic, minced

½ tsp dried rosemary

1 tsp chili powder

1 cup beef stock

1 cup heavy cream

1 onion, chopped

1 tbsp olive oil Pepper

Salt

## DIRECTIONS

1. Add oil into the instant pot and set the pot on sauté mode.

2. Add rosemary, garlic, onion, and chili powder and sauté for 5 minutes.

3. Add meat and cook for 5 minutes.

4. Add remaining ingredients and stir well.

5. Seal pot with lid and cook on high for 30 minutes.

6. Once done, allow to release pressure naturally for 10 minutes, then release remaining using quick release. Remo e lid.

7. Serve and enjoy.

**NUTRITION:** Calories 575, Fat 29g, Carbs 4.3g, Sugar 1.3g, Protein 70.6g, Cholesterol 244mg

# Mouth-Watering Lamb Stew

**Servings:** 4

**Preparation time:** 180 minutes

## INGREDIENTS

- ½ cup golden raisins

- 1 cup dates, cut in half

- 1 cup dried figs, cut in half

- 1 lb lamb shoulder, trimmed of fat and cut into 2-inch cubes

- 1 onion, minced

- 1 tbsp fresh coriander

- 1 tbsp honey, optional

- 1 tbsp olive oil

- 1 tbsp Ras el Hanout

- 2 cloves garlic, minced

- 2 cups beef stock or lamb stock

- Pepper and salt to taste

- ¼ tsp ground closes

- ½ tsp ground black pepper

- 1 tsp ground turmeric

- 1 tsp ground nutmeg

- 1 tsp ground allspice

- 1 tsp ground cinnamon

- 2 tsp ground mace

- 2 tsp ground cardamom

- 2 tsp ground ginger

- ½ tsp anise seeds

- ½ tsp ground cayenne pepper

## DIRECTIONS

1. Preheat oven to 300F.

2. In a small bowl, add all Ras el Hanout ingredients and mix thoroughly. Just get what the ingredients need and store remaining in a tightly lidded spice jar.

3. On high fire, place a heavy-bottomed medium pot and heat olive oil. Once hot, brown lamb pieces on each side for around 3 to 4 minutes.

4. Lower fire to medium-high and add remaining ingredients, except for the coriander.

5. Mix well. Season with pepper and salt to taste. Cover pot and bring to a boil.

6. Once boiling, turn off the fire and pop the pot into the oven.

7. Bake uncovered for 2 to 2.5 hours or until meat is fork-tender.

8. Once the meat is tender, remove it from the oven.

9. To serve, sprinkle fresh coriander and enjoy.

**NUTRITION:** Calories 633, Fat 21g, Carbs 78g, Protein 33g

# Beef With Tomatoes

**Servings:** 4

**Preparation time:** 40 minutes

## INGREDIENTS

2 lb beef roast, sliced

1 tbsp chives, chopped

1 tsp garlic, minced

½ tsp chili powder

2 tbsp olive oil

1 onion, chopped

1 cup beef stock

1 tbsp oregano, chopped

1 cup tomatoes, chopped

Pepper

Salt

## DIRECTIONS

1. Add oil into the instant pot and set the pot on sauté mode.

2. Add garlic, onion, and chili powder and sauté for 5 minutes.

3. Add meat and cook for 5 minutes.

4. Add remaining ingredients and stir well.

5. Seal pot with lid and cook on high for 30 minutes.

6. Once done, allow to release pressure naturally for 10 minutes, then release remaining using quick release. Remove lid.

7. Stir well and serve.

**NUTRITION:** Calories 510, Fat 21.6, Carbs 5.6g, Sugar 2.5g, Protein 70g, Cholesterol 203mg

# Lamb And Peanuts Mix

**Servings:** 4

**Preparation time:** 20 minutes

## INGREDIENTS

- 2 tablespoons lime juice

- 1 tablespoon balsamic vinegar

- 5 garlic cloves, minced

- 2 tablespoons olive oil

- Salt and black pepper to the taste

- 1 and ½ pound lamb meat, cubed

- 3 tablespoons peanuts, toasted and chopped

- 2 scallions, chopped

## DIRECTIONS

1. Heat up a pan with the oil over medium-high heat, add the meat, and cook for 4 minutes on each side.

2. Add the scallions and the garlic and sauté for 2 minutes more.

3. Add the rest of the ingredients, toss, cook for 10 minutes more, divide between plates, and serve right away.

**NUTRITION:** Calories 300, Fat 14.5g, Fiber 9g, Carbs 15.7g, Protein 17.5g

# Cheddar Lamb And Zucchinis

**Servings:** 4

**Preparation time:** 30 minutes

## INGREDIENTS

1 pound lamb meat, cubed

1 tablespoon avocado oil

2 cups zucchinis, chopped

½ cup red onion, chopped

Salt and black pepper to the taste

15 ounces canned roasted tomatoes, crushed

¾ cup cheddar cheese, shredded

## DIRECTIONS

1. Heat up a pan with the oil over medium-high heat, add the meat and the onion, and brown for 5 minutes.

2. Add the rest of the ingredients except the cheese, bring to a simmer and cook over medium heat for 20 minutes.

3. Add the cheese, cook everything for 3 minutes more, divide between plates and serve.

**NUTRITION:** Calories 306, Fat 16.4g, Fiber 12.3g, Carbs 15.5g, Protein 18.5g

# Fennel Pork

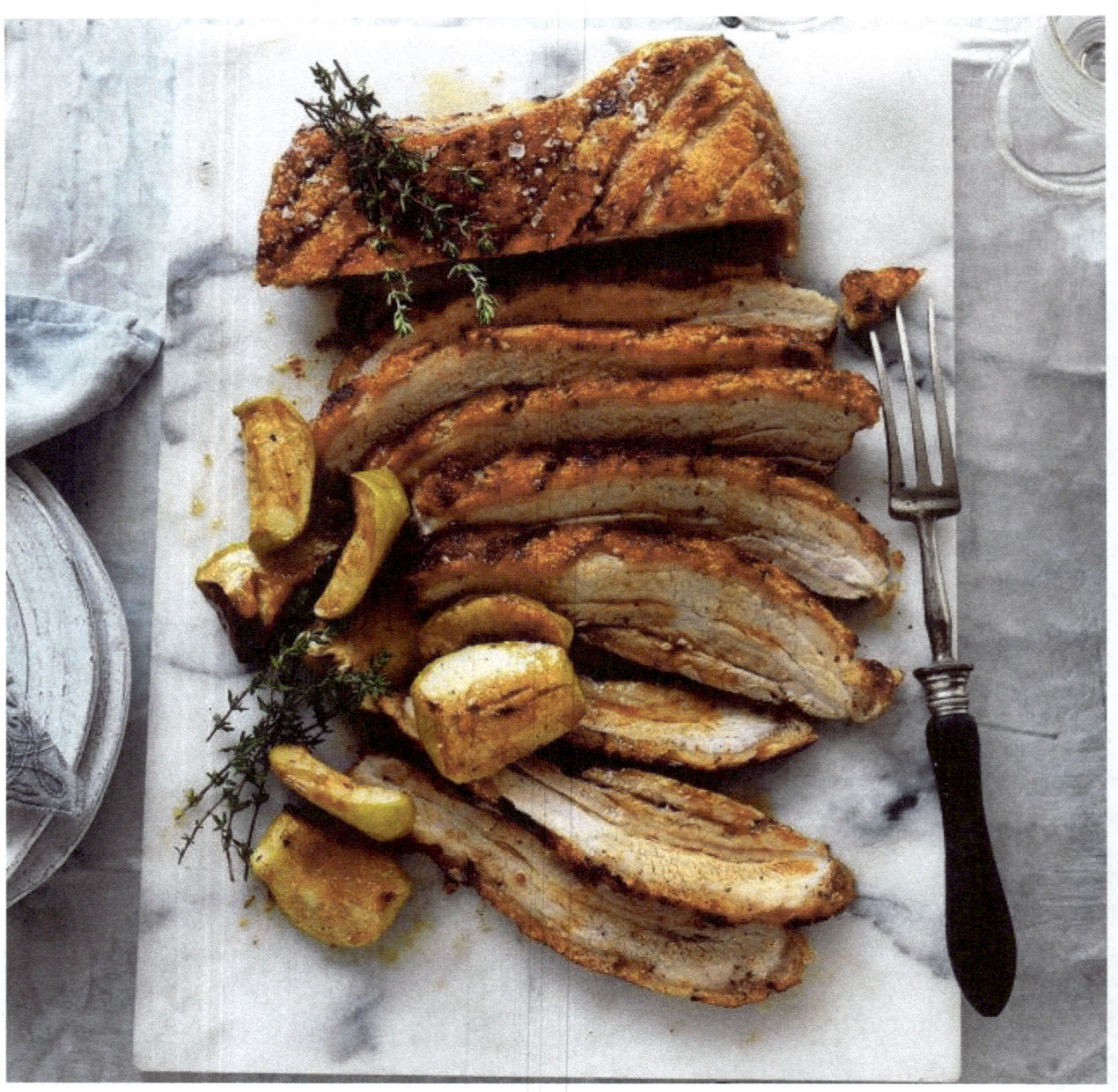

**Servings:** 4

**Preparation time:** 2 Hours

## INGREDIENTS

*   2 pork loin roast, trimmed and boneless

- Salt and black pepper to the taste

- 3 garlic cloves. minced

- 2 teaspoons fennel, around

- 1 tablespoon fennel seeds

- 2 teaspoons red pepper, crushed

- ¼ cup olive oil

## DIRECTIONS

1. In a roasting pan, combine the pork with salt, pepper, and the rest of the ingredients, toss, introduce in the oven and bake at 38 degrees F for 2 hours.

2. Slice the roast, divide between plates and serve with a side salad.

   **NUTRITION:** Calories 300, Fat 4g, Fiber 2g, Carbs 6g, Protein 15g

# Lamb And Feta Artichokes

**Servings:** 6

**Preparation time:** 8 Hours

## INGREDIENTS

- 2 pounds lamb shoulder

- 2 spring onions, chopped

- 1 tablespoon olive oil

- 3 Garlic cloves, minced

- 1 tablespoon lemon juice

- Salt and black pepper to the taste

- 1 and ½ cups veggie stock

- 6 ounces canned artichoke hearts. drained and quartered

- ½ cup feta cheese, crumbled

- 2 tablespoons parsley, chopped

## DIRECTIONS

1. Heat up a pan with the oil over medium-high heat, add the lamb, brown for 5 minutes, and transfer to your slow cooker.

2. Add the rest of the ingredients except the parsley and the cheese, put the lid on, and cook on low for 8 hours.

3. Add the cheese and the parsley, divide the mix between plates and serve.

   **NUTRITION:** Calories 330, Fat 14.5g, Fiber 14.1g, Carbs 21.7g, Protein 17.5g

# Lamb And Plums Mix

**Servings:** 4

**Preparation time:** 6 Hours and 10 minutes

## INGREDIENTS

- 4 lamb shanks

- 1 red onion, chopped

- 2 tablespoons olive oil

- 1 cup plums, pitted and halved

- 1 tablespoon sweet paprika

- 2 cups chicken stock

- Salt and pepper to the taste

## DIRECTIONS

1. Heat up a pan with the oil over medium-high heat, add the lamb, brown for 5 minutes on each side, and transfer to your slot cooker.

2. Add the rest of the ingredients, put the lid on, and cook on High for 6 hours.

3. Divide the mix between plates and serve right away.

**NUTRITION:** Calories 295, Fat 13g, Fiber 9.7g, Carbs 15.7g, Protein 14.3g

# Lamb And Mango Sauce

**Servings:** 4

**Preparation time:** 1 Hour

## INGREDIENTS

2 cups Greek yogurt

1 cup mango, peeled and cubed

1 yellow onion, chopped

1/3 cup parsley, chopped

1 pound lamb, cubed

½ teaspoon red pepper Blakes

Salt and black pepper to the taste

2 tablespoons olive oil

¼ teaspoon cinnamon powder

## DIRECTIONS

1. Heat up a pan with the oil over medium-high heat, add the meat, and brown for 5 minutes.

2. Add the onion and sauté for 5 minutes more.

3. Add the rest of the ingredients, toss, bring to a simmer and cook over medium heat for 45 minutes.

4. Divide everything between plates and serve.

   **NUTRITION:** Calories 300, Fat 15.3g, Fiber 9.1g, Carbs 15.8g, Protein 15.5g

# Pork Chops And Cherries Mix

**Servings:** 4

**Preparation time:** 12 minutes

**INGREDIENTS**

4 pork chops. boneless

Salt and black pepper to the taste

½ cup cranberry juice

1 and ½ teaspoons spin mustard

½ cup dark cherries, pitted and halved

Cooling spray

**DIRECTIONS**

1. Heat up a pan greased with the cooking spray over medium-high heat, add the pork chops, cook them for 5 minutes on each side, and divide between plates.

2. Heat up the same pan over medium heat, add the cranberry juice and the rest of the ingredients, whisk, bring to a simmer, cook for 2 minutes, drizzle over the pork chops and serve.

**NUTRITION:** Calories 262g, Fat 8g, Fiber 1g, Carbs 16g, Protein 30g

# Lambo And Barley Mix

**Servings:** 4

**Preparation time:** 8 Hours

## INGREDIENTS

- 2 tablespoons olive oil

- 1 cup barley soaked overnight, drained, and rinsed

- 1 pound lamb meat, cubed

- 1 red onion, chopped

- 4 garlic cloves, minced

- 3 carrots, chopped

- 6 tablespoons dill, chopped

- 2 tablespoons tomato paste

- 3 cups veggie stock

- A pinch of salt and black pepper

## DIRECTIONS

1. Heat up a pan with the oil over medium-high heat, add the meat, brown for 5 minutes on each side and transfer to your slot cooker

2. Add the barley, the rest of the ingredients and put the lid on, and cook on low for 8 hours.

3. Divide everything between plates and serve.

   **NUTRITION:** Calories 292g, Fat 12g, Fiber 8.7g, Carbs 16.7, Protein 7.2g

# Cashew Beef Stir Fry

**Servings:** 8

**Preparation time:** 15 minutes

## INGREDIENTS

- ¼ cup coconut aminos

- 1 ½ pound ground beef

- 1 cup raw cashews

- 1 green bell pepper, julienned

- 1 red bell pepper, julienned

- 1 small can water chestnut, sliced

- 1 onion, sliced

- 1 tablespoon garlic, minced

- 2 tablespoon ginger, grated

- 2 teaspoon coconut oil

- Salt and pepper to taste

## DIRECTIONS

1. Heat a skillet over medium heat, then add raw cashews. Toast for a couple of minutes or until slightly brown. Set aside.

2. In the same skillet, add the coconut oil and sauté the ground beef for 5 minutes or until brow.

3. Add the garlic, ginger and season with coconut aminos. Stir for one minute before adding the onions, bell peppers, and water chestnuts. Cook until the vegetables are almost soft.

4. Season with salt and pepper to taste.

5. Add the toasted cashews last.

**NUTRITION:** Calories 325, Fat 22g, Carbs 12.4g, Protein 19g

# Conclusion

We have actually gotten to completion of this wonderful yet tiny publication.

I have actually presented you to my favorite dishes, however I'll maintain publishing even more publications with even more dishes. Make certain to exercise food preparation; attempt as well as attempt once again these scrumptious dishes that are healthy as well as healthy and balanced. Constantly speak to a medical professional prior to beginning any kind of dietary strategy and also take pleasure in life. I eagerly anticipate seeing you at the following one. Delight in.

CPSIA information can be obtained
at www.ICGtesting.com
Printed in the USA
BVHW051645140521
607367BV00015B/2069